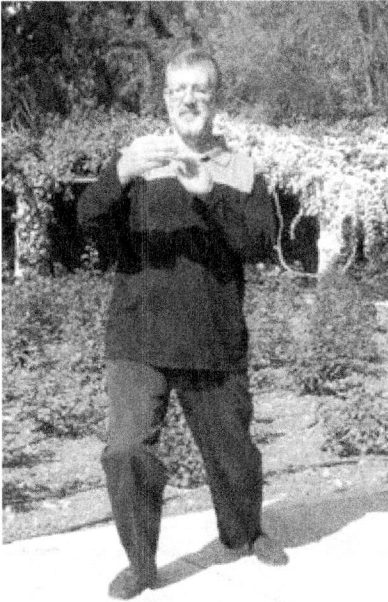

TAI CHI: DANIEL LONEY

You have been a guest on the Parkinsons Recovery radio show and even offered Tai Chi workshops on the Parkinsons Recovery Cruise to Alaska. Now you are one of the Pioneers of Recovery. How did all of this come about?

DANIEL LONEY: *Arieh Breslow who teaches tai chi was a guest on your radio show last year. Arieh has a lot of experience working with people who have movement disorders and several of his clients are people with Parkinson's. During that interview he mentioned a person by the name of Danny who had been doing Tai Chi before he developed the Parkinson's symptoms. He said that this particular person had been successful in slowing down the progression of Parkinson's and almost doing away with most of the symptoms all together. That person happens to be me. I contacted you and the rest is history.*

> Can you share with us your fascinating personal story?

DANIEL LONEY: *Yes, of course. There are two areas that I want to cover. Firstly my own personal story about how I cope with Parkinson's and how I use Tai Chi to accomplish that. And secondly, I want to discuss the Tai Chi classes that I teach for people with Parkinson's.*

Tai Chi for Parkinson's Disease

First, I will share a little about myself. I was born and raised in Oregon and at the age of 25, I immigrated to Israel with my family and three small children. Later I had one more child born here. I've been in Israel for 28 years now. I've worked in the computer industry for 35 years and I have been practicing Tai Chi for 19 years.

I had my first Parkinson's symptoms at the age of 49, about eight years after I started Tai Chi. But, Parkinson's isn't the first neurological disease that I've had. When I was 33 years old, about a year before I immigrated to Israel, I had an autoimmune disease called <u>Guillain-Barré</u> which affects one out of every 100,000 people. This disease is a result of a virus. Your body builds up antibodies to fight the virus and once the virus is gone, these antibodies begin to attack the peripheral nervous system. Within a period of a few days, a person can lose the ability to walk. It is not uncommon to have difficulty swallowing. As the nervous system

3   *Parkinsons Recovery*

deteriorates, you may even have to be put on a respiratory machine.

I didn't deteriorate to that point, but I did begin having problems with swallowing, so the doctors decided to try an experimental treatment on me. This treatment consisted of taking blood out of one arm, putting it through a machine which replaced the plasma and then pumping it back into the other arm. The entire procedure takes about five hours.

After the third treatment I started to respond and began getting better. However, part of my peripheral nervous was damaged. I was unable to walk when I was released from the hospital. As my nerves started slowly growing back, I had to teach myself to walk all over again. I used a walker and started by walking from one side of the room to the other. Then, eventually I could walk down the block and back. I kept working at it and over a period of about a year and a half I recovered with the exception of a few small symptoms that are still with me to this day.

For example, when I get tired I tend to have a little numbness in my fingers and my toes. Also I tend to have a little bit of a balance problem that is still due to the Guillain-Barré. I usually tell people I'm a neurological wreck. The Guillain-Barre took care of my peripheral nervous system. Now, Parkinson's seems to be doing a job on my central nervous system.

Most people do recover eventually but usually there is some sort of permanent damage. After recovering from Cuillain-Barre, I went back to work and pretty much led a normal life. Several years later, I started studying with Arieh, who has been my first and my only Tai Chi teacher for over 18 years now. I'll always be indebted to him for what he has taught me. He not only has been my Tai Chi instructor, but he has showed me how to

Tai Chi for Parkinson's Disease

live and how to balance my life.

I started doing Tai Chi because Tai Chi really addresses the area of stability, balance and coordination which were some of the problems that I retained as a result of the Gillain-Barre.

Tell us about your experience with Parkinson's

DANIEL LONEY: *I noticed my first Parkinson's symptoms twelve years ago. However, I was experiencing symptoms for about two years before I was diagnosed. There were some early symptoms which I ignored because I didn't know they were symptoms of Parkinson's. For example, when I was doing the Tai Chi sword form, my left arm wasn't always quite in the right place during certain moves. My brain was telling me it was but when I looked my arm just wasn't where it was supposed to be. I also noticed that when I was walking my arm didn't quite swing freely; there was stiffness in it.*

I complained to my general practitioner. He thought that it might be from the fact that I work with computers all the time and I'm on a keyboard a lot. So, we never really went into it very deeply. About two years later I started developing a small tremor in one of my fingers and then at that point I knew that something was probably wrong. I knew that I needed to see a neurologist.

So, I made an appointment with a neurologist. I remember walking into his office and before I even opened my mouth, he took one look at me and said, "You have Parkinson's. Your face is expressionless, you're stooped when you walk and you have a tremor..." At that time I just went into shock. I really didn't know exactly what Parkinson's was. I didn't understand the full implications of what he had said. He started writing out a prescription of pills; all different kinds of pills. My head was in a total haze after he said that I had Parkinson's.

After I finished with the doctor I went to meet my wife at a restaurant for dinner. I didn't say anything to her right at the beginning. We went ahead and ordered our food and after the food arrived she asked, "Well how did your exam go?" "The doctor said that I have Parkinson's." I began to explain to her what I could comprehend from the doctor's visit. One of the things the doctor did say was that the medication works well for about three years. They call this the honeymoon period. During those three years when you're on the medication you feel as if you don't have Parkinson's at all. After three years as you get worse the medication starts to lose its effectiveness and then you start to feel like you're going downhill. This I explained to my wife.

The way we interpreted the whole story was that I had about three years left. That's how I felt. I had three good years left and after that it was going to be all downhill. So of course by the time our food arrived we weren't very hungry.

I came home and looked up Parkinson's on the Internet and found a list of all the Parkinson's symptoms. There were about 20 major symptoms listed and I started going through them one by one. I had almost every single symptom. That was very, very depressing. Of course, I didn't want to believe what the doctor said on a simple walk in the door, look at me, you have Parkinson's type of thing. So of course we got a second opinion and they ran all kinds of tests, MRIs and blood tests and through the process of elimination they basically said well: you don't have this and you don't have that, you don't have this other thing, so you must have Parkinson's.

I was pretty depressed because based on the doctor's prognosis I didn't have a very bright future. I had those three good years left and that was about it.

Unfortunately, about two weeks later my mother passed away. She had an extended battle with cancer and so I had to fly back from Israel to Oregon in order to help arrange the funeral. By that time my symptoms were bad enough that I wasn't even sure that I'd be able to make the trip. However, I did make the trip and of course losing a parent is something very hard to go through and it aggravated the symptoms that much more.

On top of that, in Jewish tradition we have a seven-day mourning period that is a very heavy type of mourning where we sit in the house of the deceased and let people bring us food and serve and comfort us. But right in the middle of the seven-day mourning period was the famous 9/11 Twin Towers attack. I had planned on staying in Oregon just for the seven days then flying back to Israel and slipping back into my normal way of life. Unfortunately, all the airports were closed

Tai Chi for Parkinson's Disease

down and I wasn't able to get a flight for another two weeks. By the time I finally did make it back to Israel I was a real basket case. I was really in bad shape.

Needless to say, I went into a period of depression. I wouldn't say it was a severe depression but it was a period of depression. During that year of mourning for my mother I wasn't mourning just for her. I actually found that I was mourning for myself as well. I felt that I had been given a death sentence. I had these three years hanging over my head and then my life would be going downhill. So I was mourning for my mother and I was mourning for myself at the same time.

I began to go downhill very rapidly. My condition deteriorated till I got quite bad. I almost quit doing Tai Chi all together. In fact I wasn't able to do it. I tried doing the Tai Chi form which consists of very slow movements and I was shaking so badly that I couldn't even get through it. I

Parkinsons Recovery

stopped going to classes. I stopped taking lessons from Arieh because I was very embarrassed that the other students would see my shaking.

I also was having difficulty doing my job because I began to suffer from confusion, anxiety, and panic attacks. When I was in meetings, I would come out of the meeting many times unable to remember what was discussed. I remember going to one meeting with my partner. Our boss spent a half hour explaining to us everything that he wanted us to do. When I came out of the meeting, I said, "Abraham I think I'm losing it, I didn't understand a thing that he said in that meeting." And Abraham turned to me and said, "That's okay, I didn't understand a thing either." That incident was a pleasant reality check that I had not lost my sanity completely. Also, part of my job working with computers entails hauling around cables and plugging the cables into the back of computers and test equipment. Many times I was shaking so bad that I couldn't even plug a cable into a computer without the aid of some else. So I was in very bad shape. My self-confidence in my body was just totally destroyed. My mind was willing, but my body wouldn't do what my brain was telling it to do.

I went through a period of time, about a year, where I was seeking out various alternative treatments. I tried Ayurvedic medicine with herbs and was taking yoga lessons. I went to a Tibetan monk and received massage treatments along the various energy meridians and also acupuncture. I tried Chinese herbology; all of these helped to some extent, but not really a lot. I wasn't taking western medication at that time.

I went about three years without taking the medications. I was looking for an alternative treatment instead. Finally something happened that changed my whole approach. I'm not the type of

*person who takes a lot of stock in dreams;
I wasn't then, but now I do. One night I
had a very vivid dream of my mother. She
was crying and she was rubbing my cheek
and she was saying it's going to be okay,
it's going to be okay. I didn't really
understand what that meant. I found
various sites on the internet for dream
interpretations. So I went to one of the
sites and I found that a crying parent
usually has something to do with a
chronic illness. The fact that she was
saying it's going to be okay, it's going to
be okay, meant it really was going to be
okay. Over a period of several weeks I had
several other vivid dreams and when I
looked at the interpretations of them they
all said that my subconscious was trying
to communicate with my conscious that it
was about time to make some very drastic
changes in my life; changing directions
completely. So I knew that something big
was going to be happening.*

At that point I decided that I could spend

the rest of my life running around, traveling around the world seeking out all types of alternative treatments, spending a lot of money but nothing was going to help unless I was willing to take responsibility for myself. Western medicine wasn't going to be able to cure me or help me or relieve my symptoms. And likewise, alternative medicine wasn't going to be able to help me or cure my symptoms. It was going to be basically up to me. I could rely on western medicine and I could rely on various alternative things as well, but all in all what was really going to save me and help me was taking responsibility for my own health. Everything else would be in conjunction with that. I reached the conclusion that I had the tools all along to help myself and what I had to do was get back to Tai Chi because that's what I know, that's what I'd been studying all these years and that's what was going to be the key for dealing with my Parkinson's symptoms. And based on the dreams I knew I had to do some very serious reprioritization of my life and there was going to be a lot of changes coming.

I began by writing a list of items summarizing how I wanted to spend the rest of my life. What would make me happy and be rewarding? There were three things on my list. The first was family. I wanted to enjoy my family and to help them realize their goals and aspirations and just be with them.

The second item on my list was to build clocks. Clocks are a hobby of mine. I build six foot tall grandfather clocks. After I had been initially diagnosed with Parkinson's, I was looking for a hobby in order to help maintain my fine motor skills. I decided I would do what my father did - I would build a grandfather clock for each of my kids. So that's what I'm doing, I have one clock built now and I have just started on the second clock. I have four clocks to do all together. The first one was built from a kit but the rest of them will probably be built from scratch. When I have completed making those four clocks I will probably build a clock my wife and myself and who knows who else.

The third item on my list was to help others through Tai Chi. An item that was not on that list was work. Several days after I made my list, I went into work and I assembled my bosses. They knew that I had Parkinson's. I'd been open from the very beginning when I was initially diagnosed with Parkinson's. So I told them that it was becoming increasingly difficult for me to do my job and I was going on sick leave. I had about 6 months of sick leave accrued because I had taken very little sick leave during the years that I had worked at this company. I told them that I was going on extended sick leave and during that period of time I intended to apply for disability pension. If I did not get disability pension then I might come back. But, if I did get it they would not see me again. I haven't been back to work since.

Shortly after I "retired" or stopped working I entered the stage of life that I call Tai Chi, Tai Chi, Tai Chi. I put extreme emphasis on Tai Chi. I began taking Tai Chi very, very seriously in order to reduce my symptoms and improve my quality of life. The depression and mental symptoms disappeared almost immediately as I gained self-confidence doing the Tai Chi movements. And as I began to gain my strength back, my tremor disappeared almost completely. If you see me on the street you will not see me shaking. I'm very relaxed. I've reduced the stress in my life. Retiring from my job has been the main reason for that. My walking has improved. I no longer stoop when I walk. I walk upright. I have improved stability and coordination and much better over-all body strength. So, I was able to reduce many of my symptoms through serious involvement in

Tai Chi for Parkinson's Disease

Tai Chi over a period of about six months to a year.

Today my daily exercise routine consists of about 40 minutes of Tai Chi in the morning, walking almost every day between 30 and 40 minutes and lifting light weights two or three times a week. I don't believe in over- exercising and in running myself down. I believe that after a workout you should feel energized. You shouldn't feel overly tired. So usually an hour to an hour and a half max is my exercise routine for the day.

Do you attend a Parkinson's support group?

DANIEL LONEY: *Yes, I do. I am involved in the Israel Parkinson's Association. They have branches in all the major population centers in the country; there are 12 branches altogether and each branch has a support group. I'm very involved in a support group and we meet once every two weeks. There are about 26,000 people with Parkinson's in Israel out of a population of 7 million. I think that if you work that out statistically it comes out to about the same proportion of people who have Parkinson's in the United States.*

Tell us about your affiliation with the Israel Parkinson's Association

DANIEL LONEY: *When I was initially diagnosed with Parkinson's I had signed up with the Israel Parkinson's Association. However, because of my depression, I did not attend very many meetings. One day I got a phone call, or I should say my wife got a phone call, from the Israel Parkinson's Association. They mentioned to my wife that they were looking for a sports teacher, someone who was willing to work with Parkinson's people on some sort of exercise program. My wife told them that her husband isn't a sports teacher but he is a Tai Chi instructor, and so of course they were very interested in that.*

Tai Chi for Parkinson's Disease

I explained to the head of the Jerusalem Branch over a cup of tea that I had stopped teaching Tai Chi altogether because of my Parkinson's. I was very self-conscious of my tremors and of my symptoms and I didn't feel comfortable teaching even though I was in the process of recuperating from many of my severe symptoms. Anyway, she insisted on arranging a demonstration at the next Parkinson's meeting and I agreed.

When I arrived that evening there were 40 people there sitting around in a large circle and I was in the middle. Using my notes, I began explaining what Tai Chi is and after five minutes I kept getting these blank looks. People didn't understand. I probably wasn't explaining it correctly or it probably wasn't interesting. Maybe I was boring. I don't know. So I decided that it was time to ad-lib.

I invited my wife to join me in the middle of the circle and I said, "Okay, I want you throw a punch. This is your opportunity!!" When she threw the punch, rather than block it, I merged with her energy and as she punched, I yielded. I yielded back and drew her in so that she lost her balance. And when she came off balance, I was able to push her very lightly causing her to almost fall. Those watching thought, hey, that's really cool.

Afterwards, I went around the circle so that everyone could see and some people were getting out of their seats saying, "Do that again. Do that again." She was trying to give me a punch and I was yielding with it and coming back and pushing her very lightly, knocking her off balance. If I really would have pushed her, I could have actually pushed her up against the wall and really hurt her.

I explained to them that Tai Chi is a series of self-defense moves strung together and executed in a predefined form. Then I slowly began to do the form. I was very nervous. I was solo in front of 40 people in the middle of a circle and I had never done that before in my life. I noticed a tremor in my right hand and I was thinking to myself that they were going to notice the shaking. But then I said to myself, "Everyone in this room is shaking, what does it matter?" So I went through the first third of the form and when I finished... complete silence, nothing. You could hear a pin drop. I looked around and I said to myself, "Oh no, was I that bad?'

So then I started doing the form again and as I was doing the form the second time I started to explain the application of each position. People began to get up out of their seats and crowd around me. They were looking very closely and I started hearing remarks of, "Wow isn't that beautiful?" "The posture is unbelievable," or, "isn't that amazing." Of course, with all of the positive comments I was getting better and better at doing the movements.

When I finished doing the form the second time, I started going through it a third time explaining some of the principles; softness, relaxing, movement originating from the hips and separation of weight. I looked up and all around the room everyone was trying to copy me. People were out of their wheelchairs, people had their walkers against the wall, and even the hired care-givers were trying to do it.

It was like one big party. People were laughing and smiling. That was a high point in my life. People could really identify with what I was doing.

I then began to explain the importance of proper rooting. When you go to a neurologist, one of the first things he does is check your stability. He stands in back of you and he tells you to stand straight and he puts both hands on your shoulder and he gives you a flick and tries to pull you backwards to see if he can knock you off balance and determine whether you can regain your balance. If you stand stiff as a board you are just going to go right over.

How can you pass the neurologist's test? Pretend you are a tree with roots going deep into the ground. Your body is like the trunk softly swaying in the wind. Now when the doctor pulls you back, it will be a lot harder to pull you off balance. He still may succeed in pulling you off balance but it's going to be a lot harder. The group was amazed at this and so everyone wanted to try it. By the end of the evening, I had fourteen people who had already signed up for my first Tai Chi group.

Now that I had a group I had to decide what I was going to teach. I had never taught people with movement disorders before or people with Parkinson's. Since Parkinson's in a progressive disease, I felt that a reasonable goal would be after six months to a year of doing Tai Chi my students could come to me and say they didn't get worse. If they could at least say that they hadn't gotten worse that was already positive. I also felt that I wanted to be true to the masters, by teaching pure Tai Chi. I wasn't out to make a name for myself or to come out with a new methodology. I wanted to teach pure Tai Chi as passed down to me by the masters.

What Tai Chi exercises do you introduce in your Parkinson's classes?

DANIEL LONEY: *Well first of all, many of the exercises that I do are taken from various movements of the Tai Chi the form. I constantly create new exercises and look at new ideas. As I began to talk to Parkinson's people about other exercise classes they attended, two major complaints kept surfacing.*

First, the exercises were too difficult. Second, the instructors were not familiar enough with their needs. I knew that I had to develop exercises simple enough so that people could do them and enjoy them. If you don't have fun doing them, you are not going to do them on a daily basis. As far as understanding their needs, who better could understand their needs than someone who has Parkinson's, someone who lives their symptoms? I knew what worked for me and I was willing to share with them what I believed would work for them as well. So as I said before, I'm constantly adding new exercises. It is very creative and exciting to develop new exercises based on Tai Chi principles.

Second, many times I try to use every day experiences when I develop new exercises. For example, I developed an exercise to aid moving in crowds. One evening, my wife wanted to go to a crafts fair at a park. We got there and it was mobbed. The booths and exhibits were on grass, the ground was uneven, little kids were running around, people were jostling each other and pushing each other. I looked at the crowd from a distance and thought as a Parkinson's person that it would be suicide to go in there. But, I had promised my wife and she really wanted to go.

So as we began to walk, I said to myself that the only way I'm going to get through this is to be flexible, to pretend once again like I'm a tree, that I have my roots deep into the ground and my body is a swaying trunk. Normally, if I'm walking along and someone is walking in the opposite direction and their shoulder hits my shoulder and I remain stiff, he is going to knock me over. When I am hit or jostled I want to remain soft so that the on comer turns me like a revolving door. I turn with their hit and they glide right by me. So, that's one of the exercises that I teach - to be sensitive not only to your own body but when you are touched by other bodies, to be sensitive to their feel and their touch and their strength. You learn to yield to them and that keeps you from being pushed over.

When I started teaching my first session I did some general warm-up exercises and various coordination exercises to gauge where people were at and see what kind of shape they were in. After about ten minutes I said to myself, "Oy vey! These guys are unbelievable. There is a hand here and a foot there and a leg there and an arm there–everything is all over the place." There was no integration of the body parts whatsoever. We could not start at the beginning. We would have to go back before the beginning. We would not be able to start at zero, but would start at minus 10.

So I concentrated on doing very basic strengthening exercises and after about three months I was able to start where I would start with a normal class. Six months later when I looked at the class, and I saw how they moved, it was unbelievable. It made me cry to see the improvement that they had made. They were fluid and flexible. It is hard to believe.

I have received some really good compliments from my students. I had one lady come up to me say that before taking Tai Chi lessons, her husband refused to go out of the house because he was too self-conscious in public. But now he goes out of the house on his own for walks. In another instance, the wife of another student came up to me while we were on a walking tour with them in Jerusalem. She said, "My husband would have never gone on a tour like this before. He would not have been able to stand long enough or walk such distances, but look at him, he's out here and he's walking and he's having a good time." So Tai Chi works. It works. If you dedicate yourself to it and you practice it and you do it every day, it works. I'm convinced of that. It works for me and it works for my students.

What are the benefits of Tai Chi?

DANIEL LONEY: *I think that Tai Chi is expressly built to help people with Parkinson's. It's an all encompassing workout. It strengthens the body – by that I mean the muscles, the joints, the bones and internal organs as well. It increases your flexibility and opens your joints. Many of the exercises work on stability and balance. The exercises also work on coordination and teach your body to function as one integrated unit that moves together as a whole. In other words, when you move your arm it won't go one place and your leg another place. Everything moves as one integrated whole. It improves your posture. Tai Chi employs deep breathing so you're breathing much deeper and much more freely.*

One of the main things it does is that it increases your bodily awareness through meditation. When you are doing the form slowly, you are meditating on your body.

Tai Chi for Parkinson's Disease

You become very aware of your body and where each part is. Where's my hand? Where's my foot? Where are my hips? Are they in line? Is my head directly over my shoulders? Are my shoulders directly over my hips? Working on minute points of bodily alignment is very, very important. Also because it is meditative you reduce stress by going deep into yourself, allowing you to know yourself better. You become familiar with your strengths as well as your limitations.

Another important factor for people with Parkinson's is that it helps restore self-confidence. You are able to see that you can still do things you did not even think you could do. You can do certain things that normal people cannot do. This gives a great boost to your confidence. With a chronic illness like Parkinson's, your confidence in your body is destroyed completely. But, once that confidence begins to return you become so much happier. You are much more involved in life. You are more exuberant. You are a much more caring person willing to give of yourself.

Describe the lessons you offer in a Tai Chi class

DANIEL LONEY: *In many cases, my classes are structured as a mini-support group. I encourage everyone to talk freely. We discuss each other's symptoms, medications and ways for dealing with the symptoms. My students are not just students to me. They are personal friends. Another main ingredient of the class is that it should be fun. If the class isn't fun, people aren't going to practice the exercises at home.*

My typical class lesson consists of several components. We start out with stretching and strength exercises. These exercises are based on Tai Chi principles. Next, we do Qigong, which are Chinese medical exercises intended for various parts of the body and specific organs. These exercises tend to stress deep breathing, reducing stress and flexibility. Then we work a lot on walking. In fact, I have several walking exercises where I have people walk forward, then sideways, and then backwards. I even have a cross-step exercise using a sword. Walking is a very, very important part of the whole routine.

With the walking exercises there are also hand movements that accompany them so that we are developing coordination as well. For example, in walking forward, we pretend that we are softly weaving silk, gently pulling the silk from a cocoon. When walking sideways we become a cloud in the sky gently floating across the sky. All of the exercises have specific names usually tailored after things in nature or animals. We also work with partners. We gently push each other so that we can become sensitive to another person's energy. This assists in preventing falls and helps when moving in crowds.

Tai Chi for Parkinson's Disease

Who sponsors your classes?

DANIEL LONEY: *Most of my activities are sponsored by the Morton Apfeldorf Parkinson's Support Foundation (http://www.apfeldorffoundation.org) . This is a non-profit organization set up for the express purpose of enhancing the quality of life of people with Parkinson's.*

Most of my Tai Chi classes are offered through the Israel Parkinson's Association. I'm well known in Israel among the Parkinson's circles and I do workshops at their national conferences. I also speak to other non-profit organizations about my experiences because we've found that what works for our group often works for other support groups as well. If I had to sum it up, I would have to say that I'm extremely satisfied with what I am doing now. It is exactly what I'm supposed to be doing at this point in my life. I've learned that my life is not over because of the Parkinson's. Those three honeymoon years are long past and my life is so rewarding and fulfilling. I've never been happier than I am right now.

DANIEL LONEY: *If you want to know more about me and my services, I have a web site at www.taichiparkinsons.com. For anyone that is a Tai Chi instructor who either currently teaches people with Parkinson's or would like to teach people with Parkinson's, I would be willing to meet with them or have a telephone conversation with them. They can contact me at mailto:loney.daniel@gmail.com. I can share my experiences with them, advise or help out in any way possible.*

In addition, if you are part of a Parkinson's support group and you are interested in organizing a Tai Chi class for your support group, I can make suggestions about choosing a competent

Tai Chi for Parkinson's Disease

Tai Chi teacher. I am willing to share with the teacher and the class the types of exercises that I do and give any advice that can help you be successful.

I also usually make a trip to the States and Europe about once a year. If anyone is interested in a workshop, I'd be willing to conduct workshops for them. They can contact mailto:me loney.daniel@gmail.com. *I have already conducted workshops for a Parkinson's Recovery cruise to Alaska and for a series of support groups through the Northwest Parkinson's Association. I was also a presenter at the* World Parkinson's Congress *2010 in Glasgow.*

> What would you say to a person who has just been diagnosed with Parkinson's disease?

DANIEL LONEY: *There are several things you can do. First, get involved in a support group. Support groups are extremely important for receiving feedback from other people. You can see*

*what others are going through and what
they have experienced. Plus, they have a
lot of advice to share. I always tell people
that my heroes in life are other people
with Parkinson's. I have met incredible
people who are just normal people, but
how they deal with their Parkinson's
simply blows me away.*

*The other thing I would recommend is to
get involved in an exercise program,
whether it is Tai Chi or something else
that turns you on. Whatever it is, get
involved and make it a regular part of
your life because exercise and keeping
your body moving is one of the things that
keeps you healthy. The Chinese have a
saying that you are only as healthy as
your legs. In other words, when you lose
your legs, you lose your mobility. When
you lose your mobility, stagnation starts
to set in and that is when you become
susceptible to all kinds of diseases and
conditions.*

Tai Chi for Parkinson's Disease

Finally, and most importantly, take responsibility for yourself. **You** *need to reduce your Parkinson's symptoms yourself and you can use Tai Chi, dance, yoga, etc. to do that. Take responsibility for your health and for your future. So get moving, stay optimistic and keep a positive attitude!*

How to Hear Daniel Loney on Parkinsons Recovery Radio

Visit http://www.blogtalkradio.com/parkinsons-recovery and scroll back to find the show that aired December 3, 2009 featuring Daniel Loney as my guest.

About Daniel Loney

Daniel Loney, a certified Tai Chi instructor, has been doing Tai Chi for over eighteen years. He was diagnosed with Parkinson's disease when he was 49. After several years of physical deterioration, he was forced to retire from his job as a computer science engineer. During this time,

Daniel treated his Parkinson's symptoms using western medicine and various alternative techniques. After having only limited success in relieving his symptoms, he finally decided to take full responsibility for his health and immersed himself in Tai Chi. As a result, Tai Chi has brought Daniel sustained relief from his Parkinson's symptoms.

Today, twelve years later, Daniel does extensive volunteer work for the Israel Parkinson's Association, teaching Tai Chi classes to Parkinson's people and conducting workshops in Israel, the United States, and Europe. He was a presenter at the World Parkinson's Congress 2010 in Glasgow. He has developed an extensive repertoire of exercises based on Tai Chi principles and his unique approach has benefited many people with movement disorders.

Tai Chi for Parkinson's Disease

Printed in Great Britain
by Amazon